TURN YOUR HAPPINESS ON

TURN YOUR HAPPINESS ON

How to Light up your Days and Fill your Life with Joy

Norma Nikutowski

Turn You Happiness On:
How to Light up your Days and Fill your Life with Joy

Published by Spring Rain Publishing.

ISBN: 978-1-7326090-0-6 - paperback
ISBN: 978-1-7326090-1-3 - ebook

Printed in the United States of America

Make every day a happy day!

I dedicate this book
to everyone who is searching for a more
meaningful and joyful life.

Contents

Introduction

"Happiness is the whole aim and end of human existence."

— **Aristotle**

I grew up in Argentina in a loving family that was always concerned about safety, probably because they survived the Second World War. Our kitchen cupboards and closets were full of food cans, rice, and noodles. The front door had three different locks. The garage was full of dusty tools, gadgets, and boxes that my dad thought we might need some day. The world was scary, and there wasn't any safer place than home.

"Stay still. Be quiet."

"Don't talk unless I ask you a question."

"You got a good grade? You probably copied the answers from your neighbor."

"You got a bad grade? You did not study and for the next six months will not leave your room and study."

In my family, these phrases and comments were synonymous with "I love you."

Pointing out my every little mistake, which was a never-ending list, was a way to show their love and care. If they had not cared for me, they wouldn't have even bothered to point them out.

My most exciting trip was a once-a-week visit to the library. I loved reading about ancient civilizations and learning what it was like to live thousands of years ago in Rome and Greece, but I was most impressed by the Egyptians. In my imagination, I spent hours walking through the narrow corridors of the pyramids, considering mummification options, trying to decipher hieroglyphs, and imagining what it would be like to be Cleopatra.

In my twenties, after earning my own money tutoring students, the fantasy of visiting these faraway places haunted me daily. Despite my family's well-intentioned stories about how women travelling alone are abducted, tortured, and killed, I couldn't help myself and had to go. When I got to Cairo, I had to take a bus to the hotel. The bus was packed; there were people sitting on the floor and squeezing in every corner. The driver was nice enough to put a plastic chair next to him for me to sit on. My face was almost touching the windshield.

There was just sand and a few houses on the side of the road. In front of us, I could see a group of about ten kids and teenagers huddled close to the road. At that instant, I remembered reading that a common practice in Egypt is to throw rocks at tourist buses. I could already see a rock impacting the windshield, breaking the glass, and landing in the middle of my face along with all the broken glass. I was tense and waiting for the right second to duck beneath the windshield. I saw the kids extending their hands. Just when I was ready to hide, the hands were waving and the faces smiling. I couldn't believe my eyes. Fifteen minutes later, there were more kids along the road. Would they also wave and smile? Yes, they did. I couldn't help but wave back.

The next day, I set out to visit the pyramids in Giza. I couldn't believe I was walking in those narrow and small corridors and seeing where the pharaohs had been placed. All of a sudden, I'm surrounded by teenagers who are asking me if they can take a picture with me. With me? Why me? Were they trying to get me confused so that they could pickpocket me or steal my backpack? After a few days, I got used to people asking me to take pictures with them. It seemed that the world was not such a scary place after all.

During that trip, I clearly felt that I had "turned my happiness on." It was not about travelling or about walking inside of the pyramids; it was about doing something I had always wanted to do. After some months of sleeping in shared rooms full of strangers, taking showers in stalls without curtains, and walking around with my backpack, it was time to decide what I was going to do with the rest of my life.

So, I got my degree in psychology and worked with clients who suffered from depression and anxiety. Then, I got married, moved to the United States, became a special education teacher, and had two wonderful kids. Each of these events had "turned my happiness on," but they had happened more than ten years ago.

One morning while getting ready for work, I looked at myself in the mirror. As I do every morning, I washed my face, applied lotion, makeup, and combed my hair. I could see myself twenty years from now, full of wrinkles and white hair, repeating the exact same routine. That's when I realized, "If I don't change anything in my life right now, I will be doing exactly the same thing for the next twenty years. I am forty now; how will I feel at sixty? Happy about the road traveled, or just wondering where all those years had gone?"

That's when I started asking myself questions: Was I happy? Was I living a happy life? Was I living the life I had always dreamed about? Had I done everything I had always wanted to do? My everyday life was going to work and taking care of my family. Was that what I had always wanted to do? If there were a time to make a change, it was now. I had at least twenty wonderful years in front of me, and I wanted to really make them the best years of my life.

How do you create your best life? That's when I started to research, study, and learn all I could about happiness.

In this book, I will share everything I have learned about happiness so that you can also create an enjoyable and fulfilling life. When you look in the mirror, you will feel happy about the road travelled.

Let's "turn your happiness on."

CHAPTER 1

What Is Happiness and Where Do You Find It?

"He who is not contented with what he has, would not be contented with what he would like to have."

—Socrates

Happiness means different things to different people. Happiness is looking at the glass half-full. It's seeing the big picture, and despite emergencies, illnesses, obstacles, or other unfortunate circumstances, being able to find something to feel good about. It's seeing our problems as opportunities and having a general sense of well-being and feeling good about ourselves. It's about seeing the good qualities in ourselves and others and focusing on what we love.

How do you know if you are happy? If you feel good about yourself and your circumstances most of the time, then you are happy. For the purpose of this book, I will consider happiness as feeling good about yourself and others and having positive expectations most of the time.

The problem with happiness is that we tend to look for it in all the wrong places. Advertisements, social media, and comparisons with others lead us to believe that something new added to our lives will bring feelings of happiness. We expect that a new

- car
- house
- relationship
- beauty product
- item of clothing
- ultimate gadget
- higher-paying job
- vacation
- place to live, a different city, state, or country
- haircut
- baby

will bring more happiness into our lives. The problem is that after doing or acquiring these things and feeling ecstatic for a few weeks or months, the novelty and excitement wears off, and we go back to being and feeling like our old selves.

DOES MORE MONEY MEAN MORE HAPPINESS?

Studies[1] show that money increases well-being and happiness when it takes people from a place where there are real threats of not having enough food, a lack of safety, or crime to a place that is reliably safe. After that, money doesn't matter much. Daniel Kahneman[2], researcher and Nobel Laureate psychologist, showed that money increases happiness until people reach an income of about $75,000 annually; after that, emotional well-being does not increase with income. High income improves *evaluation of life* but not *emotional well-being*.

Emotional well-being is the emotional quality of a person's everyday experience, how often a person experiences joy, sadness, anger, and affection that make life pleasant or unpleasant. *Life evaluations* are the thoughts that people have when evaluating their own lives. Life evaluation rises steadily with higher income, while emotional well-being, as previously stated, rises up to a point of an annual income of around $75,000. Low income exacerbates the emotional pain associated with such misfortunes as divorce or illness. High income buys life satisfaction but not happiness. Low income is associated with both low life evaluation and low emotional well-being. An annual income of $75,000 is the lower limit that allows people to socialize and spend time with people they like, avoid pain and disease, and enjoy leisure activities. Income is more related to satisfaction than to happiness.

Do Your Present Activities Make You Feel Happy Right Now?

In order to increase *life satisfaction*, we keep busy, trying to accomplish an enormous amount of tasks in very short periods of time. It usually starts in the morning with the feeling that we are already late before stepping out of bed. Then we have to hurry to get ready for work, rush our significant other out the door, get the kids ready for school, and get to work on time. Once we get to work, there is a pile of things that need to be completed. After work, we are tired and just want to relax by watching TV, checking social media, e-mails, and the last trending YouTube videos. This was my everyday routine for many years.

There was not much time to think about what made me feel good. I thought it was about working hard right now and enjoying life later. "Later" could be during the weekends, vacations, or retirement. The problem with this approach was that I was so tired during the weekends that my most exciting activity was watching movies. My biggest fantasy was that money was going to solve all of my problems, and it would open a magic door where all my dreams would come true. What were my dreams? I wasn't even sure about that, but I was hoping for a magical life. I was certain that once I turned my yearly income into my monthly income, my confidence and self-esteem would soar. I imagined going to any store and choosing items without looking at the price tag. With plenty of money, I would just focus on what I loved and made me happy. So, I worked longer hours, had part-time jobs, applied for higher-paying jobs, and had more stress, but was still hoping that more money would transport me to happiness ever after. However, after many years of this routine of working like crazy, chasing money, and working myself to exhaustion, it became apparent that I was just spinning my wheels.

A few months ago, some of my octogenarian relatives passed away. They had amazing plans for their retirement and actually had the money to fulfill their wildest dreams. Did they do it? No, they spent their days watching TV, clipping coupons, shopping, and eating out. I could see myself in their shoes.

At work, people were retiring. They were ecstatic because they had worked very hard all of their lives to enjoy their retirement. They had plans for luxury vacations to exotic destinations, and for the first time, they would have time to do what they had always wanted to do. Every year for the holiday season, they came back to say hello, so I got updates on their awesome retirement lives.

Some travelled to different states to visit family. Most of them were helping their grown-up kids, watching their grandkids, and staying at home. As time went by, they started worrying about safety and health and ended up not even wanting to travel or go anywhere far from their homes. Talking to retirees year after year was an eye-opening experience. I could see myself, after a whole life worrying and chasing money, retired, sitting on the couch just worrying about my safety and health.

This made me think about my own experiences. I remembered how much I enjoyed travelling to faraway places during my summer vacations. I backpacked because it was the cheapest way to travel. I was still a student, and I wanted to see the world with my own eyes. I visited many places in America, Europe, Africa, and Asia. It was an exciting experience. It was very interesting meeting people from different cultures and seeing how they lived. It was interesting to see how quiet or busy the streets of some cities were compared to others. Now, if someone would tell me today that they would pay all the expenses for me to go backpacking to any country of my choosing, I would say, "No, thank you very much."

Even though it was an amazing experience in my twenties, I don't feel like sleeping on trains, hitchhiking, or eating tuna fish every day because the cans fit in my backpack and are easy to open. Even though I have very fond memories of that time, I don't feel like doing that kind of travelling in my forties.

This led me to think that experiences we crave today may be

totally different from our circumstances ten, twenty, or even thirty years from now. Right now, exotic vacations in Cambodia sound exhilarating, but in twenty years, Hawaii may feel more appealing, or maybe even a local beach. So, I decided that I really needed to find out how to lead a happy life while enjoying everything life has to offer and doing the things I am interested in doing *right now*. In twenty years, I will most likely be drawn to different experiences.

TURN YOUR HAPPINESS ON

The *set point theory of happiness* suggests that our level of well-being is determined by heredity and personality traits developed early in life; as a result, our happiness level remains relatively constant throughout our lives. Our level of happiness may change temporarily depending on life events, but sooner or later it will return to the baseline as we get used to those new events.[3]

Researchers at Northwestern and Massachusetts University compared the level of happiness of lottery winners and the level of happiness of patients with spinal-cord injuries. They concluded that after one year, the thrill of winning the lottery will wear off, and the accident victims will bounce back to their previous happiness level[4]. This means that it's not one big event that will shape our level of happiness or unhappiness forever after; it's the little, everyday experiences that will increase our enjoyment of life.

Every human being has the capacity to feel happy. We come into this world with our genes programmed to a certain happiness level. But this "set point" amounts to only 60 percent of our happiness. The other 40 percent of our happiness will depend on how we live our lives.

This means that we all have the capacity to feel happiness; it's just a matter of turning it on and keeping it on.

Experiences such as talking to a good friend, enjoying our favorite food, or watching our little one joyfully playing will increase our happiness level. Coming home after an exhausting day at work and finding that our dog chewed our favorite shoes, our little one got hurt, or that our significant other is grumpy will decrease our happiness level. Positive and negative circumstances alternate constantly, and so do our moods. How do you stay in a good mood despite your circumstances? How can you feel happier more frequently and for longer periods of time?

If we keep doing what we have always done, we will get the same results we have always created. If we continue running around like crazy, we will continue to feel exhausted and stressed out at the end of the day. An accumulation of stress can even create illnesses or impact our relationships with our loved ones.

To start our journey to "turn our happiness on," we need to focus on ourselves. If we are happier, people around us will also be happier.

We only have this present moment to live. It's up to us to make it a wonderful or a miserable moment. Wait a minute. Is that up to us? Are we responsible for the annoying clients who don't stop complaining or the boss who keeps making unreasonable requests, such as wanting a last-minute report and presentation for tomorrow with the promise of a promotion he has been tempting us with for the past year? How do you make it a happy moment after an exhausting day at work? We go home planning on finishing the report and watching some TV before going to bed only to find out that our little one is crying because he was pushed to the ground at school, and not only that, but he has been bullied at school for many months. So, how can it be up to us to make these miserable moments wonderful?

FOCUS ON WHAT YOU LOVE

A friend of mine who is a single mom of two teenage girls insists that their watching movies that show women being kidnapped, raped, or abused is good preparation for teaching them not be too trustful of others, especially men. She is very worried that someone may take advantage or try to hurt her young daughters, so she is trying this strategy to open their eyes about strangers. I talked to her, explaining that she may be conditioning her daughters to be too fearful or to have negative expectations about their environment. She defended her position, saying that she just wanted them to be aware that bad things can happen and that they have to keep their eyes open all the time to make sure nothing bad happens to them. I tried to explain to her that focusing so much on the negative would create more negative expectations in her daughters, but I was not able to convince her. As parents, we want the best for our kids—to be safe, to make good choices, and to make sure they will be able to provide for themselves in the future and become independent adults.

It is not always easy to focus on what we love and makes us happy because negative events are amplified by the news. We have a tendency to discuss our problems more or what is not working than what is working. People around us will contribute to our happiness depending on their positive or negative attitude.

ACTION STEP

Make a list of ten goals that you have already accomplished. You may have baked a birthday cake for a family member, completed a class, helped someone else meet a deadline, got the job you wanted, finished reading a book, exercised twice a week for a month, and so on.

1. ______________________________

2. ______________________________

3. ______________________________

4. ______________________________

5. ______________________________

6. ______________________________

7. ______________________________

8. ______________________________

9. ______________________________

10. ______________________________

BLAMING OUR PAST

My mind is mostly busy with the well-being of my kids. I think about what they like, how to help them feel safe and confident. I read books every day with both of them. We usually have some gardening, hiking, or child-centered activity during the weekends. Despite all of my efforts, my kids regularly complain that I don't pay enough attention to them.

Most of my clients complain about their dysfunctional childhoods where parents divorced, were not always present when they were needed, compared them constantly with more successful siblings, misguided them into wrong decisions, or did not realize when to stop when correcting them. Usually, parents do the best they can to raise their children. They may transmit their own frustrations and shortcomings. They don't want their kids to repeat their same story, so they go out of their way to protect them.

Unfortunately, dysfunctional parents seem to be the norm. Most parents had the best intentions and did the best they could to educate us. *Being mad about our past or thinking and rethinking about our past will keep us anchored in our past.* Every time the past comes to mind, forgive your family and relatives because they did what they considered appropriate given the circumstances. We cannot choose what type of family we are born into. Every family has some positive and negative aspects. Regardless of our upbringing and early family relationships, we cannot change our past. Dr. Wayne Dyer used to say that he was thankful to grow up in orphanages because that made him a better psychologist. Most parents do the best they can given their particular circumstances. Many abusive or neglectful parents had difficult childhoods themselves and are just repeating a cycle of dysfunction. The best thing to do is to forgive them. They probably loved us to the best of their abilities, and now it's time to move on with our lives.

However, many times, we repeat the same thinking and behavior patterns as our parents or significant others; in fact, most of our behavior derives from our significant others. We copy and emulate their behaviors, or we do exactly the opposite. If our parents had a negative outlook on life and would criticize our every move, we will most likely be very critical with our children. If we had very strict parents who would never allow us to have fun, we might be more relaxed and laid-back parents who do not put strict limits on our kids. Parents have the best intentions, but they don't always know how to phrase something or act in a positive way.

For many years, I worked with children with emotional disturbances from elementary to high school, and my overall conclusion was that if I had gone through any of the traumatic experiences that these students had, I would have been labeled emotionally disturbed, too. I've also seen the progress they made from elementary to high school—how these students were able to work themselves out of their emotional issues with mental health and school counseling. Some students were able to take responsibility for their own lives and circumstances and make the best of it, while others kept complaining about their poor circumstances and start in life.

Oprah Winfrey, twice Oscar-nominated actress and TV mogul, was sexually abused by her nineteen-year old cousin when she was only nine years old. She was also molested and severely beaten by other relatives as well. Many successful people had less than ideal families growing up but they were able to move beyond their traumatic experiences.

Thinking candidly about our past and family will help us to move on with our present lives instead of blaming our parents or our past. As human beings, we tend to blame our past for our current circumstances. We think if we had been born into a more affluent family, we would not have to struggle to make ends meet because they would have guided us to make better decisions in life, and they might even have helped us out financially. If our parents had not divorced, we would be more trusting in our relationships. If our dad would have been more loving, we would be more understanding and patient with our kids. Again, parents usually do the best they can given their upbringing and life experiences.

It's not always easy to escape from our past. It seems to haunt us when we least expect it. Before deciding to move forward in a relationship, we remember all the times we were rejected. Before applying for a job, we remember all the previous jobs we applied for and didn't get. Before deciding to change careers or start a new project, we remember all the times that we did not finish something we started in the past and all the criticism and questions that followed. We want to be successful, but we keep remembering our bad experiences in our past. We don't want to get hurt or make the same mistakes twice; that's why we remember all these negative situations so that we won't make the same mistakes again.

A good strategy to help us let go of our negative past is to focus on positive experiences. When were the times you were successful?

ACTION STEP

Make a list of five positive relationships with friends, relatives, siblings, teachers, coworkers, mentors, or pets. Think about these trusting and caring relationships.

1. ____

2. ____

3. ____

4. ____

5. ____

HAPPINESS IS AT YOUR FINGERTIPS

As newborns, we came into this world full of gifts and talents waiting to be developed so that we could grow and share them with the world. As we grew, these extraordinary skills were budding in our everyday life and activities. Look at a toddler or child; he or she is full of talents and abilities. Children are able to focus only on what they like and enjoy. As kids grow older, there are more demands placed on them, and different experiences will shape their identities and personalities. Kids adjust to their environment, so depending on what environment they grow up in, they will have more or less possibilities to develop their talents and skills. A variety of experiences during our childhood and adolescence will shape our personalities, and in some cases, inhibit our most intimate interests and skills. Then, adults start comparing us with other kids. Are you the smartest kid in class who always knows the answers? Or, are you average, good at some subjects while not so good at others? Or, are you always struggling to meet the minimum requirements to get to the next grade? Some kids are just not interested in school, and no matter how wonderful the teacher is, the interests and skills of some kids will not develop in the classroom.

My two little ones at home remind me every day about what happiness is all about. When things are very quiet around the house, I know that they are doing something they are very interested in. So, I tiptoe to my daughter's room to find her desk full of empty glue bottles, saline solution, corn starch, baking soda, glitter, beads, and food coloring. My daughter and son are so absorbed in mixing the different ingredients in bowls and trying to make slime with the right consistency and stickiness that they don't hear or see me. Their sweatshirts and faces are full of glitter, glue, and cornstarch. Each child is trying to make the perfect shade by mixing different food coloring.

I feel like reminding them that they will have to clean up the mess after they are done. I already know that they will say, "We will clean it up, Mommy." They will use a whole roll of paper towels and smear the glue with the saline solution with the food coloring and glitter all over the floor and desk and make an even bigger mess than before, and say, "We're done." I know I will end up cleaning up the whole mess. This is an example of how when we are kids we just focus on what makes us happy. Many times, I tried to convince my kids to buy all those exciting different types of slime so that they could play with them right away, and of course, hoping I would not have to clean up the mess afterward. But they insist that it is as much fun to make the slime as it is to play with it once it's done.

Watching my kids reminds me of my own childhood and all the things I liked to do. There was no slime when I was little, but I liked:

- dancing
- drawing
- playing with my pets
- exploring the plants and little creatures in the backyard
- spending time with friends
- reading
- writing
- experimenting in the kitchen
- listening to music
- going to new places

Not surprisingly, thirty years later, these are the same things that still make me happy. When I'm not in a good mood, I spend some time gardening, talking to a friend, playing with my dog, or reading a book. Doing any of these activities immediately puts me in a better mood. But we don't have to wait to be in a bad mood to do any of the things that we enjoyed when we were kids. I make sure that I spend some time every day doing at least one activity that makes me happy.

It's not always easy to distinguish among what makes us happy, what we think should make us happy, and what others tell us will make us happy. As we grow older, it becomes more confusing because we barely remember what used to make us happy. The following Action Step will remedy this situation.

ACTION STEP

Take some time to think about what you enjoyed doing at school, at home, with your friends, or alone when you were a child?

You may clearly remember two or three activities, but keep thinking about them until you come up with at least ten.

Activities that made me happy as a child or teenager:

1. __________
2. __________
3. __________
4. __________
5. __________
6. __________
7. __________
8. __________
9. __________
10. __________

Keep this list handy, as we will come back to it later.

The first strategy to increase your daily happiness level is to incorporate an activity you love into your daily schedule. Make sure you plan for it and anticipate it with joy.

Before you begin your activity, make it your intention to really enjoy it. For instance, I love cooking and trying new recipes. I always loved spending time in the kitchen with my mom. It was a very special moment because while I was peeling potatoes and she was chopping onions, I could talk to her about anything. It was a time when we were close enough together to let our minds flow while at the same time not having to stare at each other. Our hands were busy washing, peeling, or chopping while we could speak our minds in a very informal way. Nowadays, I repeat the same activity with my daughter. I have to constantly remind myself to really enjoy it because I tend to want to finish quickly, and I get upset when water drips on the floor, or peels end up on top of clean plates, or the counter gets all messy. Although I love cooking and spending time with my daughter, almost daily I have to remind myself to enjoy this activity. I have to remind myself to make it enjoyable. I think how to best organize the different tasks to minimize the mess and increase the enjoyment. Most days, our cooking together is a happy experience. When it's not, I think about what I could have done differently to make the experience more enjoyable for both of us the next time.

Think about your daily activities. How could you enjoy them more? Is there any daily task that you love doing, but as you are rushing, trying to keep everything clean and quickly finish it, you feel like it is just one more chore to complete? I have found that scheduling more time to complete certain tasks makes them more relaxed and enjoyable, and if something goes wrong, there is enough time to fix it.

ACTION STEP

We need to find happiness every day. Think about your daily routine. Do you like walking your dog, cooking, going over the mail, eating out, preparing a healthy and yummy snack, reading a good book, organizing your documents, or watching a movie? How could you enjoy them more? Make a list of daily activities that make you happy so when you are in a bad mood or have had a very stressful day, you can pull out your list and decide how to end your day on a happy note.

Everyday activities that I enjoy the most:

1. ______________________________

2. ______________________________

3. ______________________________

4. ______________________________

5. ______________________________

6. ______________________________

7. ______________________________

8. ______________________________

9. ______________________________

10. ______________________________

EXPECTATIONS

In our society, graduating from college is considered the beginning of our awesome lives, but this is just an illusion. After college, many graduates take any job they can find. This can be especially difficult in a recession or when the economic situation is unstable. The jobs they would like to find are those closely aligned with what they studied in college or graduate school. However, most graduates are forced to take any job just to pay their bills and student loans. As they need more money, they work longer hours or add second jobs. Once they get their heads above water and start feeling a little better, they get married and have kids. Now they have even more responsibilities and less time to consider their own interests, abilities, and possibilities.

The need to earn money or pay bills can also create confusion about our genuine interests. We might have been encouraged to get a part-time job just to pay some bills. Then, we need or want more money and increase the number of hours we work. At the beginning, it seems like a good idea because more money gives us access to more experiences. We keep increasing the hours we work, thinking that even more money will create even more happiness. Before we know it, we are in a trap—working countless hours, just making ends meet, in a job we highly dislike. This is definitely not a recipe for happiness.

In the next chapter, we talk more about these detours to happiness.

CHAPTER SUMMARY

- If you feel good about yourself and your circumstances most of the time, you are happy.
- Studies[5] show that money increases well-being and happiness when it takes people from a place where there are real threats of not having enough food, a lack of safety, or crime to a place that is reliably safe. After that, money doesn't matter much.
- Focus on the people, places, things, and experiences that you love. Do as many things that you love right now and plan for the near future.
- Forgive yourself and others for past bad experiences.
- Only you know what makes you happy. If you are not sure, try different activities and see how they make you feel.

CHAPTER 2

Detours to Happiness

"Anyone who has never made a mistake has never tried anything new."

—ALBERT EINSTEIN

You are exactly where you should be. The mistakes or bad decisions you made previously don't matter now. We cannot change our past, but we can create our present and future. This is what this book is about—creating a present and future of happiness and positive feelings despite what might happen. We can only control ourselves. There will always be circumstances we cannot change.

Consider the parents whose only child was killed by a drunk driver. Instead of complaining, they started an awareness program to prevent drunk people from driving to make sure it does not happen to other children and parents.

A mom of a student who committed suicide because of constant bullying shared her story on social media and started a blog to tell her story and to try and stop bullying in other schools. How could you use your negative past to build something meaningful: something that will make you feel good? Trauma can be a powerful force for positive change. Death, suffering, illness or surviving life-altering accidents might act as a turning point, changing us for the better.

WHO ARE YOU TRYING TO MAKE HAPPY?

Throughout our lives, we have the opportunity to interact with many different people. Every person we come in contact with will have his or her own opinion and point of view about the world. We all see the world from our particular colored pair of glasses. The closer the relationship, the greater impact the other person or people will have on our lives.

As kids, we try to make our parents happy and proud of us. As grown-ups, in the back of our minds, we still think about what our parents would think or say if they saw us today. Many times when making decisions, we focus more on others' opinions than on our own preferences.

I tried everything to make my dad proud of me. He wanted me to be an accountant, so I took many electives related to business and accounting, but I never really liked them. My dad adored math and science. He thought that only smart people studied these subjects. According to my dad, people who "don't have much brain" focus on social studies or humanities.

I had a pretty good biology and chemistry teacher. I enjoyed learning about animals, the human body, and chemical reactions. During my last two years of high school, my favorite subjects were biology and chemistry. The results of the vocational tests I took suggested that I pursue a career in the sciences. My dad was ecstatic. I decided to study chemistry.

As I said, I was never really good at math, but I was determined to do whatever I needed to do to get my degree. I had a math tutor during most of my high school years, so I decided that I could also have a math tutor for those math classes in college I was struggling in. I decided to get the ugliest classes out of the way first. So I studied really hard, hired tutors, and passed all those difficult math classes. I had no clue why math was so important, but I was able to mechanically solve the problems and get credit for the classes. I had rigorous routines of study. Once I passed all the math classes, I was ready to have fun with chemistry, or so I thought.

However, as it turned out, it didn't matter how hard I tried, I was always more interested in human reactions than in chemical ones. But I kept taking those chemistry classes and barely passing them and never got to the point of being interested or enjoying the process. My goal was to get that chemistry degree and make my dad happy.

I wondered, when would I start to enjoy and really be interested in learning? I had passed all the chemistry classes, but I still did not care much about how oxygen and nitrogen combined. At that point, I realized what a great high school teacher I had who had gotten me so interested in science and how bad my college professors were in comparison. My instructors were consummate researchers but awfully boring teachers. After finishing my assignments, I read self-help books trying to find and fix what was wrong. Most of the books emphasized the importance of determination. Yes, I was determined. I had gotten all the math and chemistry classes out of the way. I was going to college every day, taking the right classes and making progress.

If I were doing all the right things, why wasn't I happy? Life was supposed to be fun after high school, after passing all the boring classes, but why was it still not fun for me? I was never learning for fun; I was always studying because that was what I was supposed to do.

When I talked to my classmates, I realized how much passion they put into their work. I decided that I wanted some of that passion to rub off on me. So I joined study groups and spent a lot of time at the library discussing different class topics. While I enjoyed those discussions, I always felt like a fish out of water. At this point, I knew that I did not enjoy chemistry classes, and my life as a chemistry student would continue to be pretty much the same as it was so far. Was that something to look forward to? Not really. I had always thought that you needed to enjoy what you do. Besides my midmorning coffee, there wasn't much I was enjoying at this point.

I came to the conclusion that chemistry was not my thing. Now what should I do? I was ashamed of spending so much time and effort on something only to realize that it was not working out and would never work out. I had been doing what I was supposed to do, but it did not make me happy.

To make matters worse, well-intentioned friends and relatives advised me to continue. "You only have a few more classes, get it done." "Don't be a quitter." "Don't let your mind distract you." "If you don't finish this degree, you won't finish any other. It's about being determined." I could hear the whirlwind of voices in my mind. Was I a quitter? Didn't I try hard enough? Did everyone feel the same way? Was enjoying learning about something an unrealistic expectation?

I kept asking myself, what do I like, what do I enjoy? I looked around in my room and it was full of books. Yes, I definitely loved books. Then I looked through some of the titles; most were novels or self-help books. Yes, I loved novels and self-help books. But after reading many self-help books and going for counseling, I came to the conclusion that I was not going to make my parents happy no matter how hard I tried.

Then, I started to ask around about what other people thought I was good at. I was good at massaging my aunt's painful back, but thinking about a career in physical therapy made me cringe. I was good at baking and cooking, but I wasn't sure that being around food all day long was something I wanted to do. I loved trying different hairstyles and makeup, so I took a summer job at a beauty salon. I liked the job but had horrible back pain from standing up for so many hours.

I had read and been told many times that if you put your mind to something, you could make it happen, but what would make me happy? It seemed I was good at many things, but they were not necessarily a way to "turn my happiness on."

My biggest fear was spending two or three years working toward something only to conclude again that it was a mistake. I wanted to make the right decision this time. Asking around ended up not being really helpful because now I was more confused than before. I decided to work with a counselor to guide me in the right direction.

The counselor asked me to list all the possible career options I was considering and write the pros and cons for each option. Then, I had to number the pros and cons from one to ten, ten being the most favorable and one the least favorable. I ended up with two choices, literature and psychology. My past interactions with literature teachers had not been very positive as they usually interpreted characters and plots in very complicated ways. I loved just reading for fun. If I liked a book, I kept reading; if I did not like a book, I just put it down. There was a myth in my family that psychologists deal with crazy people, and they believed that psychologists ended up crazier than their patients. At that time, I was also attending a writing workshop, and one assignment was to go to a mental health hospital to look for someone to use as a character in one of our stories. I was very scared to spend time with institutionalized patients who had severe mental dysfunctions. But my friends encouraged me, and I ended up going. After a few minutes of walking through the hallways and talking to some patients, I was fascinated by the interesting characters I met. After that visit, I was 80 percent certain I would enjoy learning more about how the human mind works.

While my chemistry classmates were getting their first professional jobs, I was starting all over again getting my degree in psychology. After some teasing about my own mental health, my dad and the rest of the family ended up accepting that psychology was an interesting subject to study. Looking back, it was one of the best decisions I made in my life.

I share this experience as an example of how difficult it is sometimes to make a decision that will make us happy. Circumstances and well-intentioned people may steer us in a direction that does not have any meaning for us. If you keep asking yourself what you love and what makes you happy, you will make the right decisions for yourself.

ACTION STEP

Identify the person in your life whom you admired and always tried to make happy and do anything to please. This is usually a